# PURE Vulnerability

*... a powerfully authentic and uplifting TEDx talk about recovery through mental illness, reframing trauma and the journey to find wellbeing, belonging and hope*

*Kevin Snyder* (signature)

*Thank you!* (signature)

Printed in the United States of America
ISBN 978-1-956543-07-0 softcover
ISBN 978-1-956543-18-6 hardcover
ISBN 978-1-956543-19-3 e-book
ISBN 978-1-956543-20-9 audio

Book Design by CSinclaire Write-Design LLC

WRITEWAY
PUBLISHING
Raleigh, North Carolina

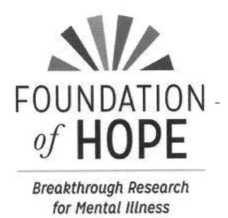

*To Mom and Dad.*

Your unconditional love saved my life.
I love you.

⌒

*To my kids, Isla and Ashton.*
You can't even read yet, but this book is for you one day.
I know there will be pitfalls and struggles
I cannot protect you from.
You are greater and stronger than any adversity you face.

⌒

*To my wife.*
I absolutely love you and what we have created together.

⌒

*And to YOU, the reader.*
However this book got into your hands,
just know it wasn't by accident.
I wish a book like this existed when I was growing up.
You're not alone.

*~ Kevin*

# PURE VULNERABILITY

# vulnerability (noun)*

*vul–ner–a–bi-li-ty*

- being exposed to openness or susceptibility of attack or harm
  *"conservation authorities have realized the vulnerability of the local population to drought and floods."*

- willingness to risk being emotionally hurt or show emotion or to allow one's weaknesses to be seen or known
  *"the foundation for open communication consists of honesty, trust and vulnerability.*

*\*from Dictionary.com*


# pure vulnerability (verb)*

*pure-vul–ner–a–bi-li-ty*

- being powerful, authentic, and courageous
  *"the pure vulnerability of what they shared was inspirational and showed strength."*

- having no fear of judgment in the spirit of helping others
  *"the openness of their story exemplified pure vulnerability."*

*\*from Kevin Snyder -- "verbalize" pure vulnerability by putting it into action for the good of yourself and others:*

# Important Note to Reader

I wish a book like this one had existed when I was growing up.

As a kid and even as a young professional, there were so many times when I felt alone. Different. Like an imposter. I encountered challenge after challenge over the years. I held in all the emotions and uncertainties, keeping everything buried inside. As an adult, I never wanted anyone to know about my past struggles, so I maintained my secrets.

Then, unexpectedly, I was moved to speak out about these challenges. And by speaking out, I mean speaking to students in classrooms. Then I was invited to speak to larger audiences. Strangers. Often I was terrified. But amazingly, using my voice to share my story turned out to become a powerful breakthrough for me and, much more importantly, for the people listening to me. I know because over and over, they have told me so.

It was my recent TEDx talk, my second talk on the TEDx stage, that inspired me to write this book. Immediately after this talk, audience members approached me, asking if the text of the talk was available somewhere. The talk was intensely personal to me, so I decided not to share the script. Several factors weighed in on that initial decision, not the least of which was how I scripted the talk was not exactly how I delivered it on stage. Once I was on stage, the audience's reaction to what I was saying took me by surprise almost immediately. Responding to the audience, I shifted what I was planning to say, opening up even more. I became emotional several times during my talk. For these reasons, I just did not feel comfortable about sharing my text upfront.

But then on the eight-hour drive home, my wonderful, supportive wife convinced me otherwise. We'll leave it at that. She's always right anyway.

Inside this book you will read the *script* for the speech with the message I intended to convey in my TEDx talk titled *Pure Vulnerability*. The message in *Pure Vulnerability* has been 30+ years in the making. Although I've presented over 1,500 times to over 1,000,000 people, my TEDx talk at Cape May was going to be the most important talk I have ever given. I didn't want to fumble it for all the right reasons—I wanted to inspire and connect with others who are struggling like I did so many times.

No pressure, right? Wrong. It was incredible pressure that I placed on myself, but it was worth it. It forced me to go to places I had never been before.

This same TEDx talk also inspired a tailored version of my bestselling book, *Think Differently to Achieve Success,* into an additional teen version, crafted and written specifically for the teenage and young adult reader. Both the adult and teen versions of *Think Differently* dive deeper into the stories and the context of the stories that I briefly addressed in my talk.

While both my TEDx talk and *Think Differently* are motivational and uplifting, some content reveals raw, vulnerable, and sensitive stories. Reader and listener discretion is advised up front.

When some chapters feel tough to read, just keep in mind that life is tough too—at any age.

I hope this book and my talk create safe spaces for us all to talk more about our struggles, our past, and our pain. Stigmas can be broken down by using our voices.

In my talk, this book, and *Think Differently*, you'll read about my experience being diagnosed with depression and an eating disorder at just 12 years old.

Fast forward to 16 when I was arrested for shoplifting. I've dedicated a short story about this experience too.

Against much recommendation, I also pushed forward and chose to write and share a sensitive and vulnerable chapter revealing my experience at 23 of being drugged and sexually assaulted by another man. Reader discretion is advised although what I have written or spoken about is not explicit.

I hope this book and my TEDx talk inspire hope in others. Regardless of how life and circumstances currently feel, I believe there is always perspective to find that can help us and others deal with those challenges. I'm living proof that you can find a way through adversity. But it's not easy. And at times, I still struggle.

Life can really suck sometimes and feel unfair. Don't ever feel alone or hopeless though. Together we are stronger.

I also hope that this book empowers you to dream BIG and think beyond the norm like never before.

I believe you can battle through any adversity to live a dream. I'm living proof. I lived my dream when I won BIG on *The Price Is Right* television game show, and I've dedicated an entire chapter to that experience in *Think Differently*. It isn't the winning that makes this story important, it's the dream around the experience that is the true story. You have dreams to make happen too.

Growing up all I wanted was to fit in and be normal. I discovered much later in life that normal doesn't exist.

Now I aspire to think differently. I strive to live in pure vulnerability.

# INTRODUCTION

I swung for the mental fences in my TEDx talk. I wanted my talk to be so raw, vulnerable, and revealing because it was finally time to share it all. The TEDx stage would be the perfect place to do so.

If you're not familiar with TEDx talks or TED talks, I encourage you to get familiar with them. In these talks, presenters share their insights, revelations, and discoveries with the general public, typically in under 20 minutes. Thousands of TEDx talks are available on both TED.com and YouTube, and hundreds have been watched millions of times. It's truly a remarkable platform for "ideas worth spreading"—the TED motto.

I shared my script for this new TEDx talk with a few close friends and asked for feedback. Consensus surprised and concerned me that perhaps my talk was "too much" in one sitting to process. Specifically, many recommended that I should cut out the story about my sexual assault and/or the campfire and/or the story about Kelly because that content on its own was a lot. They said each story could easily be its own separate and unique talk.

While I agreed in some respects, I also wanted one talk where I could land it all. No holds barred. All out. The only issue I was concerned about was keeping it close to 20 minutes.

So I trusted my gut and took a risk, making my stories concise and focusing them on the overall "idea worth spreading" embedded within my talk. I included everything I felt called to share. And for your benefit, I hope my speech was worth revealing things that I never had before.

As a professional speaker for 20+ years and presenting to over 1,500 audiences around the world, I've learned that in order to connect with an audience you must be "real." They must feel they can immediately trust you. In order to trust you, your responsibility is to be authentic, transparent, and relevant in content while also dynamic and engaging in delivery. You have nothing to sell; rather, only content to share. A great way to integrate all these elements is by crafting it all together into a powerful story.

The greatest speakers are the greatest storytellers.

I believe we all have a story inside of us and a talk idea worthy for the TEDx stage. Most people will never share theirs though. I hope this book sparks positive change empowering people to share their story or stories more often. Stigmas exist because of silence. Using our voices, we can break through the stigmas by breaking through the silence.

And when we share our story with intention to help others, we give our story new meaning. Purpose.

Nothing has meaning except the meaning we give it. So when we're able to reflect on our past and learn something from it that can be used to help others, we're better for it.

I decided to share my most difficult stories in one TEDx talk because I felt that by doing so I could help others so much better and on a bigger scale. The message embedded in my talk did not arrive to me through just one experience. It came to me through a series of events that I had kept hidden inside for far too long. And to be honest, the dots are still connecting even as I write this.

For all the right reasons, I hope you'll share my talk with others who need to hear the message I deliver. I am not alone. You are not alone. The more we talk openly about our past struggles and express pure vulnerability, the more we realize that none of us is alone.

Yes, in my normal professional speeches, I sometimes mention my depression diagnosis at just 12 years old. I sometimes mention my eating disorder too. Much less frequently, I've mentioned being sexually assaulted at 23. But that audience has been rare and only been high school or college male audiences.

Never have I had the platform to share it all in one place during one presentation and align it with one central theme and purpose . . . until my recent TEDx speech.

Preparing my speech was extremely difficult and, at times, exhausting. I had to mentally go places and reflect in ways I never had before. Being 46 years old now and revisiting things that happened when I was 12 or 16 or 23 was not fun.

It was a painful undertaking to open up my teenage diary and read about how I used to feel about myself. But it was needed in order to curate a special speech delivering the impact I intended. And by forcing myself to walk my talk of pure vulnerability, I was able to connect dots that I never had before.

I knew I would invest considerable time, so I logged all the hours I dedicated to outlining my talk, researching, scripting, practicing, editing, practicing again, editing again, etc. I hit the century mark two days before the speech went live on the TEDx stage, so I easily dedicated over 100 hours for this talk. The time doesn't matter. But to some people, especially my fellow speakers and other aspiring TEDx'ers, I feel compelled to share my time investment because a TEDx talk is not your normal speech.

Also, being married now with two very young children, my perspective on many things in life has changed. My purpose has changed too. My wife and I model behavior for our children 24-7. And I believe behavior and actions are molded by mindset.

Thinking about my kids and the future struggles they will confront, I became emotional countless times just writing the script and practicing in front of the mirror or a backyard tree. My spine would tingle, and I would wipe tears away every single time. I already have wiped tears while writing this introduction too.

When you watch my talk, you'll see I couldn't hide my emotions on stage either. For all the right reasons, I hope my talk inspires emotion in you as well. My audience felt the emotion. Our connection felt special.

Another challenge I faced in preparing my talk was that I wanted my speech to be perfect . . . which is dangerous for any presenter, because no speech is ever perfect. I've never delivered a perfect speech. Something always goes different or unexpected.

But here's the thing . . . only the presenter knows if something didn't go according to plan. As I say many times to my speaker coaching clients, *"The audience will never know it unless the presenter shows it!"*

When it comes to any speech in front of any audience, I always expect the unexpected. So I knew when I was preparing my TEDx speech that something unique would happen on stage. However, I didn't expect it to happen so immediately.

Within the first 30 seconds, my audience reacted in a way that I never anticipated. It rattled my mind from the very beginning, and I shifted my speech accordingly. Again, when you watch my talk, you'll see.

Or hopefully, you won't notice a darn thing.

I share all this context with you because 46 years of life experience has been distilled into a brief book and a short speech. I'm revealing aspects of my depression, eating disorder, arrest, and sexual assault in one sitting that might be a horse pill to swallow for some of you. Each topic and life experience could be its own book or Netflix series.

But this is also why I wanted to write a book you could consume in just one sitting. Reading this and watching my talk is not the point. What you do with the message is.

If the idea behind my talk is actually worth spreading, I hope you will join me to ignite further conversation. We need to be doing more about mental health. Especially about mental health for adolescents and young adults.

Consider how you can become a messenger along with me. Later in this book, I have shared ways to watch my TEDx talk with others and have provided discussion questions to help spark conversation.

I am honored you've taken the time to open this book, and I am hopeful my stories and insights will inspire and empower you in some way.

Here's a list of what you will find in this book:

- My original TEDx talk script
- A video link to watch the talk
- Ideas to watch the TEDx talk in group settings
- Resources available
- Important acknowledgments

I wish a book like this existed when I was growing up.

# THE TEDx TALK SCRIPT

# Pure Vulnerability

## My story and recovery from depression, an eating disorder, and sexual assault

Below is the actual script from my most recent TEDx talk that inspired this book. I wrote the script in a conversational tone. At the end of this chapter is a link to watch me delivering the message on stage. How I wrote the speech is not how I ended up delivering it.

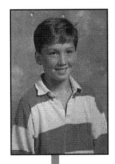

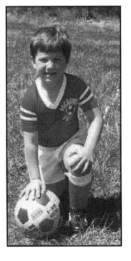

I grew up in a loving family and was a happy young kid.

But at age 12, I was diagnosed with depression and an eating disorder called anorexia nervosa.

A couple things happened earlier that year . . . a girl I *really* liked not only broke up with me, she had her friend tell me in the middle of the school cafeteria. I still remember what felt like the entire cafeteria laughing at me. Soon after, I found out she and my best friend had been dating behind my back.

I skipped school and soccer practice several times the next few weeks, because I felt embarrassed and hurt and confused.

After our soccer team lost a few big matches, coach got real mad at me and kicked me off the team, adding I had gotten fat and was out of shape.

Within a few weeks, I lost my girlfriend, my best friend, and the sport I loved—everything that meant something to me as a 12-year-old boy. I felt rejected and out of control, and I blamed it all on my weight— what I felt I could control.

I started off just wanting to lose a few pounds, but I ended up actually gaining weight. I didn't know how to diet. So after months of failure and frustration, I took a different approach and basically stopped eating and started compulsively exercising.

This is when my preoccupation with food and depression began to set in. Nights were the worst, lying in bed with insomnia and my mind racing about counting calories, push-ups, and sit-ups. I even started thinking about suicide.

This picture is from my 8th grade school yearbook. I was 5 foot 4 and 76 pounds. I had lost over 30 pounds in less than two months. You cannot tell, but I'm hiding four shirts under that sweater. You can see the bones in my face and thinning hair though.

This picture was taken just one hour before Mom pulled me out of school and took me to the doctor, again, who this time huddled with other doctors for hours because he had never treated an adolescent boy like me.

This was the 1980s, and he thought anorexia only impacted girls. The doctor told my mom I might not survive.

I am alive today for two reasons: (1) the unconditional love of my parents and (2) professional counseling.

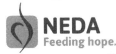

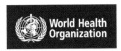

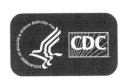

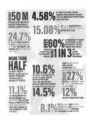

I am in front of you today to share a small part of my story from a boy's perspective of experiencing depression and anorexia and, more importantly, how I discovered a new approach living with my past as a now grown man.

According to the National Eating Disorders Association, the World Health Organization, and the CDC, the increasing rates of childhood anxiety, depression, and suicide are an urgent public health crisis. Suicide is the second leading cause of death among both adolescents and young adults, and depression is its most significant factor. Of the estimated 20 million people in the United States alone with an eating disorder, one in three is now male.[1]

We're living in a silent mental health epidemic that will not go away . . . unless we do more about it.

---

1   https://www.nationaleatingdisorders.org
    https://www.who.int/news-room/fact-sheets/detail/adolescent-mental-health
    https://www.cdc.gov/tobacco/campaign/tips/diseases/depression-anxiety.html

As I received immediate treatment and gained back some of the weight to survive, I appeared to be a "normal kid" on the outside. I felt anything but normal on the inside. I wanted to be normal so bad.

I started hanging out with new friends who accepted me, but they made bad group decisions.

Drugs. Stealing. Sneaking out of the house in the middle of the night up to no good. (Sorry, Mom, ☹, who is probably hearing this for the first time.)

We were at a store one time, and everyone was stealing things. I was the only one who got caught.

Long story short, I was arrested for shoplifting.

When school found out, they suspended me. My arrest even earned a front-page headline in the school newspaper—*"SNYDER'S SON GETS ARRESTED!"*—because my mom worked at the same school.

Now the **shame** I felt was about the embarrassment I caused my family.

Luckily graduation was just around the corner, and I could move away to college and have a clean slate, right? Yeah, right.

I struggled the first year of college . . . didn't get along with my roommate, didn't feel like I fit in, and depression creeped back in.

I tried dropping out several times, but the Dean of Students, who was required to sign my Withdrawal Form, always motivated me to keep trying and not quit. He listened to me and really seemed to care. He would say, "Give me just two more weeks before you make a life-changing decision you might regret."

Since my grades were decent, he encouraged me to get more involved on campus and meet people. One of the organizations I joined was a fraternity. At our annual campfire retreat, one of the brotherhood activities around the fire was to pull out a random card, read the question on the card out loud, then answer it.

When it was my turn, the card I pulled out was,

## "What are you most proud of?"

My answer: "I'm most proud of . . . not–killing –myself."

Then, in a moment of pure vulnerability, and for the very first time, I shared my story about battling depression, my eating disorder, and being arrested . . . *with a bunch of guys I barely knew*. I expected them to kick me out of the group.

That evening and in the days that followed, many of my new brothers approached me one to one, thanking me for sharing my story, giving me chest bumps of affection—a true sign of brotherly love. Several also shared their own struggles and mental health challenges they were no longer wanting to hide.

I soon discovered that **what I assumed to be weakness that would distance us became the strength, belonging, and bond that connected us.**

> "What I assumed to be weakness that would distance us became the strength that connected us.

After this, my entire college experience transformed, and I developed incredible friendships. My grades got even better, and I loved every minute of it all.

But probably most importantly, I stopped trying to be NORMAL. I realized normal is like chasing a ghost. It doesn't exist. One thing I learned in college is . . . Ain't No One Normal.

None of us are normal because we are all unique.

I graduated with a degree in marine biology . . . obviously. But what I really wanted to do was work in Student Affairs at a college campus. I wanted to be just like the Dean of Students who cared about me and be in a position where I could help other struggling students.

But then something happened out of the blue that changed everything . . . and my depression creeped back in.

*(Listener/reader discretion is advised)*

I was 23 years old and in my first job. The incident occurred one evening while I was visiting the home of an older work colleague who had invited me over for dinner.

He said his wife and kids were out of town for a soccer tournament. We grilled tuna steaks and asparagus and had one strawberry daquiri.

He slipped a drug in my drink that knocked me out. I woke up several hours later on his couch with my pants OFF and him ON TOP of me.

Beginning to realize he was sexually assaulting me while I was passed out, I kicked him off. Initially he said I had just had a bad dream. Then he changed his tune and said I had assaulted him.

I looked for the closest escape exit and jumped off the balcony of his second-floor condo to get to my car. As I drove off, I remember feeling so dirty, weak, and angry, as if I should have been smart enough and strong enough to prevent it.

I never pressed charges because, like most sexual assault victims, I never wanted anyone to know.

I carried this shame and kept my past hidden over the next decade while I worked on several college campuses.

I taught courses and earned a doctorate degree, the highest credential in my profession.

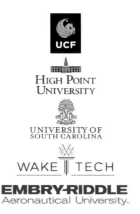

Ironically, my research was based on qualitative interviews listening to the stories of students who persevered through adversity. Achieving my dream, I was proud to have become a Dean of Students at a prestigious private university.

Along my journey, whether my student conversations were in the classroom, my office, or during my research interviews, I heard so many all-too-familiar stories about their painful struggles with anxiety, depression, belonging . . . and shame. I listened with empathy, because I understood.

While I was fascinated by the strength in their pure vulnerability, I also felt like a hypocrite for never sharing mine. I was still struggling myself.

Then yet again, something happened out of the blue that changed everything. I was invited to speak at a college leadership conference to talk about my research findings. In another unexpected moment of pure vulnerability during my speech, like the fraternity campfire, I felt compelled to share my story.

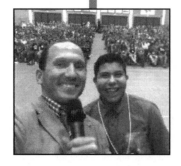

In an audience of over 1,000 strangers, I talked about my depression, eating disorder, being arrested, and even the sexual assault.

I expected them to "boo" me off stage and for the meeting planner who hired me to ask for their money back. Instead, students waited in line to talk with me afterwards, thanking me for sharing my story, some hugging me, many in tears sharing similar stories and finding strength in no longer feeling alone.

At the back of the line was one young woman in tears who said to me, "Dr. Snyder . . . I'm Kelly . . . thank you . . . I . . . " and then she ran away. I could not have stopped her if I tried.

Checking email messages the next morning, I noticed one with the subject line, "Girl who ran away." Click! It was Kelly.

She first admitted being forced to attend my speech . . . (gee thanks) . . . but then explained why.

She too was battling depression, an eating disorder, and was recovering from sexual abuse.

Kelly wrote that the only reason she had attended the conference was to kill herself. Her plan was to take her life while everyone else was attending my speech, because there would be no one in the hotel room to stop her.

But a classmate unexpectedly returned to their hotel room for a forgotten item, jokingly reminding her my speech was mandatory and literally pulling Kelly out of that room, unknowingly saving her life.

Simply connecting to the pure vulnerability of my story, Kelly no longer felt alone. She found hope, strength, and the will to finally get treatment.

After that conference I reflected quite a bit on how I could share my story beyond the classroom. As crazy as it might sound, I quit my dream job as a Dean of Students to pursue a new dream of professional speaking.

To date I've spoken for over 1,000,000 people in more than 1,500 audiences in all 50 states and several countries. I'm humbled to have presented to over 500 schools, colleges, and universities. I've also published several books, two of them being bestsellers, *Think Differently* and *PAID to $PEAK*.

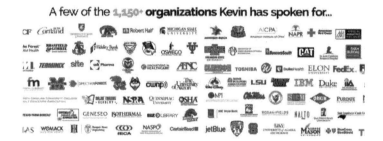

A few of the 1,150+ **organizations Kevin has spoken for...**

When people write me or come up and talk with me after a speech, usually it's not thanking me about my leadership framework or about how to be a better student, boss, or employee; rather, they thank me for helping them realize how to be a better human.

Through it all, here's what I've discovered . . . *we cannot just forget and **move on from something negative that's happened in our past** like we might so desperately want to at times.* We can only ***move forward with it*** *and perhaps even **use that experience for good*** *to help others.*

> **"**We cannot forget and ***move on from*** our past; we can only ***move forward*** by using our experiences ***to help others.***

*This is how we make (+) change. This is how we give our past new meaning. **This is how we give our pain purpose.** And I believe this is an idea worth spreading.*

So as you think about any struggles, pain, or trauma you've experienced or are experiencing that might weigh on you sometimes, just know you are not alone. In fact, you are resilient because your success rate persisting through that adversity at this point is 100%!

**Or perhaps the struggle** impacting others resulted from an action you took or inaction because you didn't do something and *that* experience weighs on you to this very moment.

Either way, I urge you to consider asking yourself *how* you can use *that experience* to help others for good in some way.

We are not better because an experience just happened to us; we are only better because of how we move forward with it.

I'm now a blessed husband and a father to two amazing young children I know will face challenges I cannot protect them from. I often wonder what their mindset will be like when they are 12 years old. Will they suffer like I did?

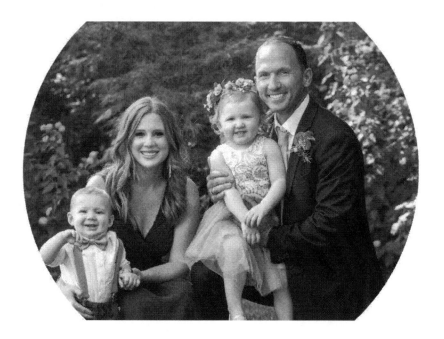

Recently, I was cleaning my attic and found the diary I wrote in while going through my depression and anorexia. Instead of throwing it away, I read it. And it was difficult.

I'd like to share with you a poem I recently wrote using excerpts from that journal and show you how I reversed it to think differently now.

*my thinking can never be changed*
*so stop trying to tell me that*
*things can be different and hope always prevails*
*because at the end of the day*
*it's too much of a negative and divisive world*
*so I'm not going to lie to you or myself by saying*
*there is hope for a better future,*
*I believe*
*that I am incapable of making a real difference*
*and nothing you say will persuade me*
*I have made too many mistakes in the past*
*I just don't believe the nonsense that*
*my past struggles have developed strength*
*because when I look in the mirror,*
*can my thinking really be any different?*

**Now reverse it and read the poem, line by line,
from the bottom back up to the top.**

I can't change or move on **from** my past, but I can choose to *think differently* about how to **move forward** with it . . . for good . . . to share my story and help others.

I believe we can all think differently. Will you join me?

# THERE YOU HAVE IT

There you have it. The planned script for my talk. Now, I would be honored if you would watch the talk that I actually delivered on the TEDx stage. It's not the same as the script.

To watch and share, visit **www.PureVulnerability.com**

or search for

*"Pure Vulnerability TEDx talk and Kevin Snyder"*
on Google or YouTube.

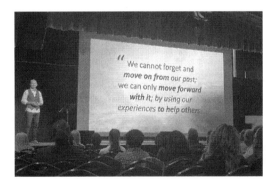

Many people have asked about the reverse poem I wrote and delivered at the end in that speech. Perspective is important in life. I have given the poem to you on its own standalone page following. The message is so important for each of us.

# TODAY I CHOSE TO THINK DIFFERENTLY

*a Reverse Poem by Kevin Snyder*

*my thinking can never be changed*
*so stop trying to tell me that*
*things can be different and hope always prevails*
*because at the end of the day*
*it's too much of a negative and divisive world*
*so I'm not going to lie to you or myself by saying*
*there is hope for a better future,*
*I believe*
*that I am incapable of making a real difference*
*and nothing you say will persuade me*
*I have made too many mistakes in the past*
*I just don't believe the nonsense that*
*my past struggles have developed strength*
*because when I look in the mirror,*
*can my thinking really be any different?*

Now reverse it and read the poem, line by line,
from the bottom back up to the top.

*Accompanying piano piece titled "Morning Hope"*
*in the TEDx talk was composed by Kevin C. Snyder ©2022*

# • BE A RIPPLE •
## IDEAS FOR GROUP SETTING DISCUSSIONS

# GROUPS

Below are ways you can leverage the Pure Vulnerability TEDx talk to spark important conversation with any group and format.

This talk introduces several topics and concepts that will benefit individuals as well as community groups, schools, teams, and especially families. The purpose behind this TEDx talk and this book is to open dialogue opportunities to help people not feel alone or isolated in adversity. Providing safe venues and opportunities to talk about difficult things can provide a safety net, a lifeline, or support—whatever you want to call it. It's up to us to provide those opportunities and safe discussions.

Topics addressed in this TEDx talk:

- Mental wellness
- Reframing setbacks to envision new opportunities
- Working through depression
- Surviving eating disorders
- Suicide prevention
- Building community and belonging
- Vulnerability and transparency
- Communication and openness
- Sexual assault recovery
- Conquering through feelings of shame and loneliness

If you are a student or educator, envision a school assembly or a classroom where students and educators watch this talk and powerful conversation follows from the discussion.

For parents, think about your family watching one night after dinner and then talking afterward. Or perhaps you watch it with your son or daughter struggling in ways that are talked about so openly about in this talk.

For professionals and community groups, imagine watching this talk during a staff meeting to help spark discussion on workplace wellness and motivation. Encourage your staff or team to watch the Pure Vulnerability talk on their own and come prepared to discuss at the next meeting. You can also leverage this talk to help set a tone for the year ahead and improve your engagement and culture.

Consider ways of hosting a group watch party, or recommending it, and then facilitating large or small group discussions afterward. Here are some possible watch parties groups:

- Educators at any level
- Student group meetings, classrooms, or conferences (school and college)
- School assemblies and events
- Professional staff meetings
- Leadership conferences
- Counseling groups and sessions
- Book clubs
- Meetups and networking groups
- Church groups
- Community groups such as Toastmasters, Kiwanis, and Rotary

Depending on the size of your group, consider small group discussions followed up with a large group debrief and sharing. Often small groups help open up conversation. The key with facilitation is creating a safe space where people feel comfortable to share and asking open-ended discussion questions.

These opportunities are how the Pure Vulnerability talk can be leveraged in ways to create a "ripple effect" of positive change through you, your organization, and beyond. This is how we all will make a difference together.

# NOTES

You can also invite Kevin to speak with your organization in-person or virtually to answer questions and share further insights. Kevin also has signature keynotes and workshops that he can deliver to your organization. Visit his website for details and to contact him and inquire about availability and pricing: **www.KevinCSnyder.com**

Even if Kevin cannot attend your group meeting, he'd love to hear how it went! Please send your feedback to Kevin directly: **Kevin@ KevinCSnyder.com**

Often Kevin hosts public meetings and webinars that you and others can join. Connect with him to follow and hear when he announces these group opportunities.

In the next pages of this book, you will find discussion questions for the following group settings:

- Educators speaking to educators
- Educators speaking to students
- Students speaking to students
- Workplace professionals speaking to their group
- Parents and families
- Customize your own! Inquire about help if needed at **kevin@kevincsnyder.com**.

As you read the book, watch the talk, or hold discussions, I invite you to post your comments on #PureVulnerability and in the **YouTube comment section**. Let's use our voices and our written words to break down barriers and stigmas. Be a ripple!

# GROUP DISCUSSION QUESTIONS

# Discussion Group Questions
## for Educators Speaking to Educators

*Below are sample open-ended questions.*
*Select those you feel are most helpful and relevant!*

- Thoughts about Kevin's talk?

- What are your top 1-2 takeaways?

- What connected with you the most?

- Did anything surprise you listening to his talk?

- What were some of the issues that Kevin shared during his talk?

- Why is talking about these issues important?

- Why is it difficult to talk about these issues?

- What are some of the issues our students are struggling with? How do we know this?

- How can we use this talk to help our students?

- How do *you* define pure vulnerability? Why is it important?

- What are ways we can help our students express their pure vulnerability?

- What do you feel about Kevin's pursuit of "being normal" and what he finally realized?

- What are ways we can deal with life when things don't necessarily go our way?

- What are resources we can take advantage of when we just want to talk with someone?

- What are resources we can take advantage of when we feel sad or are struggling?

- What are resources our students can take advantage of when they feel sad, angry, or are struggling?

- How do we ensure our students know about these resources?

- Why is it important to talk about things that are difficult to talk about?

- What can we do to help someone else who we think might be struggling?

- What are you most proud of?

- As shared in his story around the campfire, what "sparked" Kevin finding belonging and community in college?

- What are ways we can create more belonging as a class, school, or community?

- What did you feel about Kevin's reverse poem? Would you like to watch the poem again?

# Discussion Group Questions
## for Educators Speaking to Students

---

*Below are sample open-ended questions.*
*Select those you feel are most helpful and relevant!*

- Thoughts about Kevin's talk?

- What are your top 1-2 takeaways?

- What connected with you the most?

- Did anything surprise you listening to his talk?

- What were some of the issues that Kevin shared during his talk?

- Why is talking about these issues important?

- Why is it difficult to talk about these issues?

- How do *you* define pure vulnerability? Why is it important?

- What are ways we can express our own pure vulnerability?

- What do you feel about Kevin's pursuit of "being normal" and what he finally realized?

- What are ways we can deal with life when things don't necessarily go our way?

- What are resources we can take advantage of when we just want to talk with someone?

- What are resources here at school on campus we can take advantage of when we feel sad, angry, or are struggling?

- Why is it important to talk about things that are difficult to talk about?

- What can we do to help someone else we think might be struggling?

- What are you most proud of?

- As shared in his story around the campfire, what "sparked" Kevin finding belonging and community in college?

- What are ways we can create more belonging as a class, school, or community?

- What did you feel about Kevin's reverse poem? Would you like to watch the poem again?

# Discussion Group Questions
## for Students Speaking to Students

*Below are sample open-ended questions.
Select those you feel are most helpful and relevant!*

- Thoughts about Kevin's talk?

- What are your top 1-2 takeaways?

- How can we apply these takeaways in our own culture here?

- What connected with you the most?

- Did anything surprise you listening to this talk?

- What were some of the issues that Kevin shared during his talk?

- Why is talking about these issues important?

- How do *you* define pure vulnerability? Why is it important?

- What are ways we can express our pure vulnerability?

- What do you feel about Kevin's pursuit of "being normal" and what he finally realized?

- What are ways we can deal with life when things don't necessarily go our way?

- What are resources we can take advantage of when we just want to talk with someone?

- What are resources we can take advantage of when we feel sad, angry, or are struggling?

- Why is it important to talk about things that are difficult to talk about?

- What can we do to help someone we think might be struggling?

- What are *you* most proud of?

- As shared in his story around the campfire, what "sparked" Kevin finding belonging and community in college?

- What are ways we can foster a safe space where people feel comfortable to share?

- What are ways we can create more belonging here?

- What did you feel about Kevin's reverse poem? Would you like to watch the poem again?

# Discussion Group Questions
## for Professional Teams

*Below are sample open-ended questions.*
*Select those you feel are most helpful and relevant!*

- Thoughts about Kevin's talk?

- What are your top 1-2 takeaways?

- How can we apply these takeaways to enhance our own culture here?

- What connected with you the most?

- Did anything surprise you listening to this talk?

- What were some of the issues that Kevin shared during his talk?

- Why is talking about these issues important?

- How do *you* define pure vulnerability? Why is it important?

- What are ways we can express our own pure vulnerability?

- What do you feel about Kevin's pursuit of "being normal" and what he finally realized?

- How might that relate to imposter syndrome or not feeling good enough as a professional?

- What are ways we can deal with life when things don't necessarily go our way?

- What are resources we can take advantage of when we just want to talk with someone?

- What are resources we can take advantage of when we feel sad, angry, or are struggling?

- Why is it important to talk about things that are difficult to talk about?

- What can we do to help someone we think might be struggling?

- What are *you* most proud of?

- As shared in his story around the campfire, what "sparked" Kevin finding belonging and community in college?

- What are ways we can foster a safe culture where everyone feels a safe space to share?

- What are ways we can create more belonging here?

- What did you feel about Kevin's reverse poem? Would you like to watch the poem again?

# DISCUSSION GROUP QUESTIONS
## FOR PARENTS AND FAMILIES

*Below are sample open-ended questions.*
*Select those you feel are most helpful and relevant!*

- Thoughts about Kevin's talk?

- What are your top 1-2 takeaways?

- What connected with you the most?

- Did anything surprise you?

- What were some of the issues that Kevin was open about?

- Why is talking about these issues important?

- What can we do as a family so everyone feels safe to talk openly?

- What can I be doing better as a parent to make sure you feel safe talking openly?

- How do *you* define pure vulnerability? Why is it important?

- What did you think about Kevin's pursuit of "being normal" and what he finally realized?

- What are ways we can deal with life when things don't necessarily go our way?

- What are resources we can take advantage of when we just want to talk with someone?

- What are resources we can take advantage of when we feel sad, angry, or are struggling?

- What are *you* most proud of?

- As shared in his story around the campfire, what "sparked" Kevin finding belonging and community in college?

- What did you feel about Kevin's reverse poem? Would you like to watch the poem again?

# DESIRE KEVIN TO SPEAK?
# NEED HELP OR DESIRE FEEDBACK
# FOR SMALL GROUP FACILITATION?

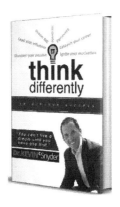

Dr. Snyder is a certified trainer, facilitator, and keynote speaker. He can help you design group facilitation curriculum or deliver one of his engaging keynote presentations, either in-person or virtually.

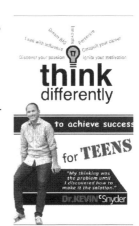

Most commonly, he is invited by schools and professional organizations to keynote at various types of events:

- School assemblies
- Faculty/staff events
- Educator activities
- Conferences and events of all types
- Half and full day employee development events
- Retreats

Inquire with Kevin about your needs, and we will explore how to help. Visit **https://www.kevincsnyder. com/hire-kevin/** where you can share more about your event!

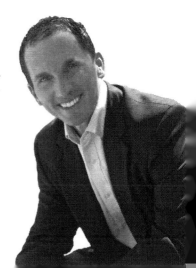

# THINK DIFFERENTLY TO ACHIEVE SUCCESS

Kevin's books, *Think Differently to Achieve Success* and the tailored version for teens, *Think Differently to Achieve Success … for TEENS*, both dive much deeper into the stories Kevin shared in his TEDx talk in their own dedicated chapters inside the book.

Despite the natural assumption of these issues, stories, and topics being difficult to read, Kevin writes about them in the spirit of an honest and uplifting tone. Both versions of *Think Differently to Achieve Success* are inspirational books comprised of stories and chapters on personal motivation, leadership, teamwork, and "dreamwork."

Inside these books you'll also read more about how Kevin lived his dream of being on *The Price Is Right* television game show and why this is an important story. This is the story that forms his signature keynote speech and launched his professional speaking career.

*Available where most books are sold*
*and on Kevin's website, www.KevinCSnyder.com*

**Would you like:**

- Bulk order discounts
- Customized books with your organization's logo and welcome message on the inside front page
- Autographed copies

Send an email to Kevin directly
at **Kevin@KevinCSnyder.com.**

# Closing Thought

---

You and I are not alone.

Our struggles and stories connect us.

What makes us *different* also makes us *unique*.

What makes us *unique* makes us *beautiful*.

Different = Beautiful.

So Think Differently and beauty begins.

I'm honored to share my stories and insights with you.

I hope you'll share yours too.

Stigmas and assumptions exist because of silence.

Let's break the silence and honor ourselves.

*— Kevin*

# RESOURCES

# Resources

As I said in my TEDx talk, I am alive today because of the unconditional love of my parents and professional counseling.

While my parents researched and found me the help I needed, I believe it was talking to a professional mental health counselor privately that helped me deal openly with my silent pain and recondition my mindset to beat depression and my eating disorder. Professional counseling is also what I relied on after my sexual assault experience.

My parents struggled finding me the help I needed because male anorexia and depression was so rare in the 1980s. The doctors didn't know what to do with me. Our family insurance initially didn't even cover my treatment. I remember my folks tirelessly talking with doctors and others trying to figure out how to get me the help I needed. So I realize that it can be confusing and overwhelming knowing where to start to get help.

I am not a medical professional. My doctorate was earned in Educational Leadership, so the information following is not about providing medical advice or treatment advice. However, based on my own experience as well as the experience with countless others, professional counseling must be a top treatment option.

Talking to a friend is not the same as talking with a professional counselor. Granted, talking about struggles to anyone is helpful, but a licensed professional such as a psychologist will know what to do and how to refer additional resources in the community if needed.

Treatment is not a one-size-fits-all approach. Professional counseling was my primary treatment option. Although some doctors tried prescribing me anti-depressants and experiential drugs, I was able to beat my depression with organic professional counseling. I never took a pill. However, I know others who do need medication while also in professional counseling.

If you're a student in any grade elementary to high school, consider talking with your guidance counselor. They are professionals who will be able to recommend resources to help you or your friend in need. Most every school has a guidance counselor, but if you're not aware of who they are, simply visit the school office and ask where their office is or ask a teacher. Guidance counselors are trained professionals and have made a career in serving students.

If you're a college student, consider talking with your Counseling Center on campus. I've spoken on over 500 college and university campuses and have worked at five. There was a Counseling Center at every single one of them. They are often located somewhere in the Student Union or near Health Services. They are usually easy to find, and services are very likely free for students. Counseling staff are trained professionals who are amazing people dedicated to listening to students in order to help them succeed.

If you're a professional at any age and employed, most companies have a wellness or employee assistance program integrated in their benefits and compensation offerings that can pay for or subsidize professional counseling. If you're unsure, simply speak with someone in Human Resources. If you find out that your benefits package does not include any type of counseling, still speak with Human Resources for any referrals in the community they might be able to provide. If you're a professional on any type of student campus, you can also ask your counseling staff for any community referrals. They cannot treat you, but they can refer you.

The following websites can be a great resource for you to find help either in your local community or on a national scale. Be careful about Googling sites and ending up going down a rabbit hole path of online noise and disinformation. Chat rooms are some of the worst. Be very careful about them. What might seem helpful for community building could lead to destructive ideas. If you do go online, start with these websites below. If you do visit online chat rooms, only visit those vetted and recommended by a licensed mental health professional.

## ANAD

National Association of Anorexia Nervosa and Associated Disorders (ANAD) is a non-profit, 501(c)(3) organization providing free, peer support services to anyone struggling with an eating disorder. (888)-375-7767. **https://anad.org/**

## Jed Foundation

Promoting emotional health and suicide prevention among college students, this website provides an online resource center, ULifeline, a public dialogue forum. **http://www.jedfoundation.org/students**

## NEDA

National Eating Disorders Association (NEDA) is the largest non-profit organization dedicated to supporting individuals and families affected by eating disorders. You can chat online with a trained professional, speak with someone or even text. If you are in a crisis and need help immediately, text "NEDA" to 741741 to be connected with a trained volunteer at Crisis Text Line. Crisis Text Line provides free 24/7 support via text message to individuals who are struggling with mental health, including eating disorders, and are experiencing crisis situations. **https://www.nationaleatingdisorders.org/**

## The National Suicide Hotline
Open 24 hours per day, 7 days per week, staffed by trained professionals. Call them at 1-800-273-8255.

## Mental Health Resources for Parents of Adolescents and Young Adults
https://www.adolescenthealth.org/

## National Institute of Mental Health
This website provides easy-to read guides and brochures to help better understand a variety of mental health disorders. **www.nimh.nih.gov/health/index.shtml**

## National Suicide Prevention Lifeline
1-800-273-TALK (8255). **www.suicidepreventionlifeline.org**

## RAINN
Rape, Abuse & Incest National Network (RAINN) is the nation's largest anti-sexual violence organization. RAINN created and operates the National Sexual Assault Hotline in partnership with more than 1,000 local sexual assault service providers across the country. If you or someone you know has been sexually assaulted, help is available. 800-656-HOPE (4673)

# ACKNOWLEDGMENTS

# ACKNOWLEDGMENTS

What I reveal inside this book as well as the book production process itself would not have been possible if not for a village of exceptional, selfless, and caring people.

First and foremost, I must honor and acknowledge my mom and dad. Without you fighting for me, I would not have learned how to fight for myself. Your sacrifice and patience with me as a teenager, and even now at times too, is a testimony to unconditional love. You saved my life on numerous occasions, and you didn't even know it.

To my older brother and younger sister. Even when I was sick, I looked up to you both. Still do. I don't remember much about our relationship during my dark times growing up, but my depression and anorexia must have been very confusing for you both, especially at the dinner table. I'm so glad our families have become so close.

To my wife. Your support and encouragement for me to share my story instilled my purpose to share it on the TEDx stage. Your patience and love are also greatly appreciated, especially when I need them the most. You're the best life coach I could possibly have and you make me a better man. I love you.

For my kiddos. Besides ensuring you feel unconditional love from your mom and me, my greatest purpose as your father is modeling behavior that will instill in you confidence, belief, and determination. Writing my speech and this book was not easy, but you made it worth it. You'll never know how much you are loved until you have children of your own one day.

To Norris Clark, Executive Director, and the incredible team at TEDxCapeMay. I am grateful for being selected as one of your speakers to share my story on your TEDx stage. Thank you for supporting and trusting me to deliver an idea worth spreading.

To my fraternity brothers at Zeta Tau Chapter and the entire Delta Tau Delta organization. My college transformation would not have been possible without experiencing brotherhood in its purest and most vulnerable form. That campfire where I shared my story for the first time was the beginning of an incredible journey, and I'm forever grateful to have such a positive fraternity experience.

To Kelly. You said I saved your life, but you saved mine. Your courage and pure vulnerability to share your story with me inspired me to share all of mine and with purpose. I would not be speaking professionally today if it weren't for you reminding me that every voice needs to be heard. I'm so proud of the great work you are doing now counseling youth.

To my 500 mastermind group. I'm always uplifted when we meet and held accountable in between. You were the first to see my reverse poem as a draft and your encouragement to share it is why I knew it was part of my TEDx idea. Thank you for the nudge.

To Kelly Swanson, my speaking mentor. I saw you speak before I met you and knew you would be a special person. Our conversations inspired me to be a better storyteller like you.

To my piano teacher. You were so cool letting me play my own music during practice lessons. I took it as a compliment when you said I played like Yanni. ☺ You inspired me to compose my own music. I hope you smile when listening to the piano behind my reverse poem.

To my 7th grade girlfriend who dumped me and my 7th grade best friend who dated her behind my back, I do not blame you. I should have made this clear in my TEDx talk. My depression and anorexia were sparked from a series of unfortunate events, adding in some puberty, hormones, and genetic disposition. In case you have figured out who you are, it's all good. Please do not feel bad. Instead, let's toast a drink at our next school reunion. First round on me.

To "Dr. Carol," my counselor. You saved my life. I can't even imagine how difficult our early counseling sessions were for you as I just sat there in silence staring at the carpet for 55 minutes. Your compassion, professionalism, and expertise helped me reprogram myself as a teenager. I would desperately need these lessons again later in life. We did this together.

To "Dean Terry," you cared enough to keep me from quitting by refusing to sign those Withdrawal Forms. Not only did you help me find the belonging and community I craved and needed so badly but you also inspired me to pursue a career and be a Dean of Students like you.

I am indebted to my editor for my TEDx talk and this book as well as the entire team at WriteWay Publishing. I doubted publishing this, but your encouragement made me think differently. I'm grateful to you and so appreciative of your expertise. More books to come I hope.

And last but certainly not least, I sincerely want to acknowledge YOU the reader as well. For whatever reason you decided to start reading this book and are reading this far to the very end, know there is something special about you. I hope my story inspires you and reminds you that you are never alone.

Ever.

Made in the USA
Columbia, SC
31 July 2023

21071657R00043